Shakespeare
on
LOVE

Shakespeare
LOVE
ON

EDITED BY

Stephen Brennan

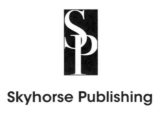

Skyhorse Publishing

Skyhorse Publishing books may be purchased in bulk at special discounts for sales promotion, corporate gifts, fund-raising, or educational purposes. Special editions can also be created to specifications. For details, contact the Special Sales Department, Skyhorse Publishing, 307 West 36th Street, 11th Floor, New York, NY 10018 or info@skyhorsepublishing.com.

Skyhorse® and Skyhorse Publishing® are registered trademarks of Skyhorse Publishing, Inc.®, a Delaware corporation.

Visit our website at www.skyhorsepublishing.com.

10 9 8 7 6 5 4 3 2 1

Library of Congress Cataloging-in-Publication Data is available on file.

Cover design by Danielle Ceccolini

Print ISBN: 978-1-62914-412-2
Ebook ISBN: 978-1-63220-122-5

Printed in China

Contents

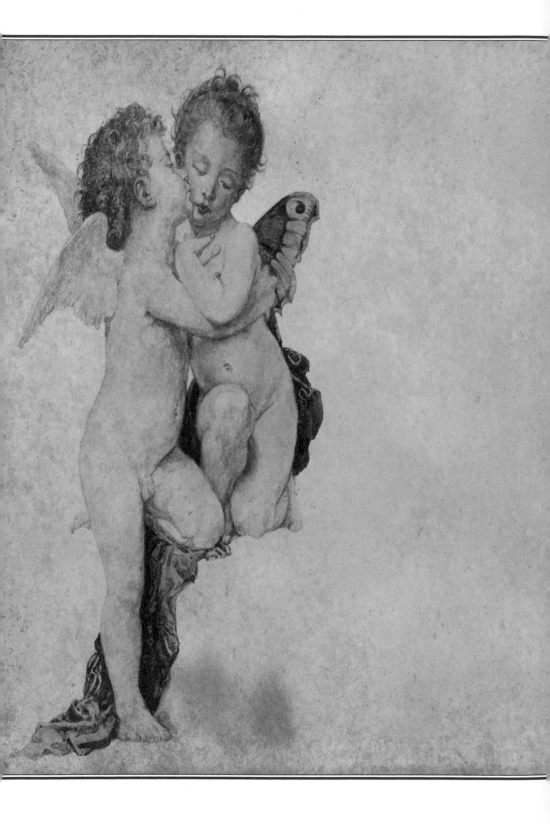

Smote
By
Love

Did my heart love till now? Foreswear it, sight.
For I ne're saw true beauty till this night.

Romeo and Juliet

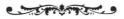

The rarest dream that e'er dulled sleep.

Pericles

O excellent young man!

As You Like It

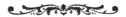

O brave new world,
That hath such people in 't!

The Tempest

O, you have heard something of my power, and so stand aloof for more serious wooing.

Pericles

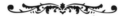

My heart itself plays "My heart is full."

Romeo and Juliet

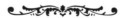

I burn, I pine, I perish,
If I achieve not this young modest girl.

The Taming of the Shrew

I do adore thy sweet grace's slipper.

Love's Labour's Lost

O brawling love, O loving hate,
O anything of nothing first create!
O heavy lightness, serious vanity,
Misshapen chaos of well-seeming forms!
Feather of lead, bright smoke, cold fire,
sick health,
Still-waking sleep that is not what it is!
This love feel I, that feel no love in this.

Romeo and Juliet

[I] dare not offer
What I desire to give; and much less take
What I shall die to want.

The Tempest

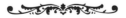

A woman is a dish for the gods if the devil dress
her not.

Antony and Cleopatra

Too fair, too true, too holy,
To be corrupted with my worthless gifts.

The Two Gentlemen of Verona

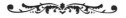

O, wonder!
How many goodly creatures are there here?

The Tempest

Thy beauty hath made me effeminate.

Romeo and Juliet

If it be thus to dream, still let me sleep!

Twelfth Night

I have night's cloak to hide me from their eyes,
And but thou love me, let them find me here.
My life were better ended by their hate
Than death prorogued, wanting of thy love.

Romeo and Juliet

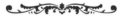

My affections
Are then most humble; I have no ambition
To see a goodlier man.

The Tempest

I love thee: I have spoke it.

Cymbeline

O wonderful, wonderful! And most wonderful
wonderful! And yet again wonderful! And after that
out of all whooping.

As You Like It

His qualities were beauteous as his form,
For maiden-tongued he was, and thereof free;
Yet, if men moved him, was he such a storm
As oft 'twixt May and April is to see,
When winds breathe sweet, untidy though
they be.
His rudeness so with his authorized youth
Did livery falseness in a pride of truth.

A Lover's Complaint

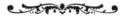

Be but sworn my love
And I'll no longer be a Capulet.

Romeo and Juliet

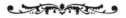

Now I will believe that there are unicorns.

The Tempest

Is it possible
That love should of a sudden take such hold?

The Taming of the Shrew

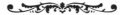

Celestial as thou art, O! pardon love this wrong,
That sings heaven's praise with such an earthly
tongue.

Love's Labour's Lost

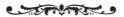

A pack of blessings light upon thy back.

Romeo and Juliet

How prettily the young swain seems to wash
The hand was fair before.

The Winter's Tale

Show pity or I die.

The Taming of the Shrew

⸻

But soft, what light thru yonder window breaks?
It is the east and Juliet is the sun!

Romeo and Juliet

⸻

When most I wink, then do mine eyes best see,
For all the day they view things unrespected;
But when I sleep, in dreams they look on thee,
And darkly bright are bright in dark directed.
Then thou, whose shadow shadows doth make bright,
How would thy shadow's form form happy show
To the clear day with thy much clearer light,
When to unseeing eyes thy shade shines so!
How would, I say, mine eyes be blessed made
By looking on thee in the living day,
When in dead night thy fair imperfect shade
Through heavy sleep on sightless eyes doth stay!
All days are nights to see till I see thee,
And nights bright days when dreams do show thee me.

Sonnet XLIII

Now heaven walks on earth.

Twelfth Night

Enchanted Tarquin answers with surmise,
In silent wonder of still-gazing eyes.

The Rape of Lucrece

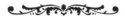

Summer hath no such a flower.

Romeo and Juliet

Run, run . . . carve on every tree
The fair, the chaste, and unexpressive she.

As You Like It

An eagle, madam,
Hath not so green, so quick, so fair an eye.

Romeo and Juliet

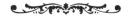

She that you gaze on so, as she sits at supper.

The Two Gentlemen of Verona

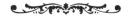

O blessed, blessed night, I am afeared,
Being in night, all this is but a dream,
Too flattering sweet to be substantial.

Romeo and Juliet

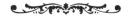

Now, at the latest minute of the hour,
Grant your love.

Love's Labour's Lost

. . . In love, i'faith, to the very tip of the nose.

Troilus and Cressida

O Romeo, Romeo, wherefore art thou Romeo?

Romeo and Juliet

Weary with toil, I haste me to my bed,
The dear repose for limbs with travel tired;
But then begins a journey in my head,
To work my mind, when body's work's expired:
For then my thoughts, from far where I abide,
Intend a zealous pilgrimage to thee,
And keep my drooping eyelids open wide.

Sonnet XXVII

Heaven's bounty . . . in you . . . beyond all talents.

Cymbeline

She's a most triumphant lady, if report be square
to her.

Antony and Cleopatra

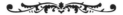

Thou wast the prettiest babe . . .

Romeo and Juliet

If you will not murder me for my love, let me be your
servant.

Twelfth Night

My heart beats thicker than a feverous pulse.

Troilus and Cressida

I have lost myself, I am not here.
This is not . . . he's some other where.

Romeo and Juliet

❧

Mine eyes,
Which I have darted at thee, hurt thee not.

As You Like It

❧

Under love's heavy burden do I sink.

Romeo and Juliet

❧

What dangerous action, stood it next death,
Would I not undergo, for one calm look.

The Two Gentlemen of Verona

By heaven I love thee better than myself.

Romeo and Juliet

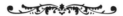

I know not why
I love this youth, and I have heard you say,
Love's reason's without reason.

Cymbeline

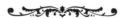

I have fallen by prompture of the blood.

Measure for Measure

The game was ne'er so fair and I am done.

Romeo and Juliet

Who ever lov'd that lov'd not at first sight?

As You Like It

He lives not now that knows me to be in love, yet I am in love, but a team of horse shall not pluck that from me; nor who 'tis I love: and yet 'tis a woman; but what woman I will not tell.

The Two Gentlemen of Verona

. . . Bewitched by the charm of looks.

Romeo and Juliet

. . . the fairest I have yet beheld.

The Winter's Tale

I am bound to wonder.

Cymbeline

⁂

Happiness courts thee in her best array.

Romeo and Juliet

⁂

In the morn and liquid dew of youth
Contagious blastments are most imminent.

Hamlet

⁂

Thou hast not loved
. . . if thou hast not broke from company
abruptly as my passion now makes me.

As You Like It

Beauty too rich for use, for earth too dear.

Romeo and Juliet

How hard it is to hide the sparks of nature.

Cymbeline

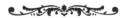

When she has obtain'd your eye,
Will have your tongue too.

The Winter's Tale

O noble stain!
O worthiness of nature! Bred of greatness!

Cymbeline

The dearest morsel of the earth.

Romeo and Juliet

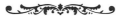

Hear my soul speak:
The very instant that I saw you, did
My heart fly to your service; there resides,
To make me slave to it.

The Tempest

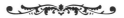

There was a pretty redness in his lip,
A little riper and more lusty red
Than that mix'd in his cheek; 'twas just the difference
Betwixt the constant red and mingled damask.

As You Like It

How angel-like . . . !

Cymbeline

O royal piece!

The Winter's Tale

What man art thou that thus bescreen'd in night
So stumblest on my counsel?

Romeo and Juliet

[She is] a gift of the gods.

Cymbeline

I hereupon confess I am in love; and as it is base for a
soldier to love, so am I in love with
a base wench.

Loves Labour's Lost

And by the way, you shall tell me where in the forest
you live.

As You Like It

This is the prettiest low-born lass that ever
Ran on the green-sward.

The Winter's Tale

I will kiss thy foot: I prithee, be my god.

The Tempest

By Jupiter, an angel! Or, if not,
An earthly paragon! Behold divineness!

Cymbeline

My bounty is as boundless as the sea,
My love as deep: the more I give to thee
The more I have, for both are infinite.

Romeo and Juliet

Skin as smooth as monumental alabaster.

Othello

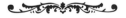

Not a heavenly saint . . . but . . . an earthly
paragon.

The Two Gentlemen of Verona

This youth, howe'er distress'd, appears he hath had
good ancestors.

Cymbeline

Shakespeare on Love

My mistress's eyes are nothing like the sun;
Coral is far more red than her lips' red;
If snow be white, why then her breasts are dun;
If hairs be wires, black wires grow on her head.
I have seen roses damask'd, red and white,
But no such roses see I in her cheeks;
And in some perfumes is there more delight
Than in the breath that from my mistress reeks.
I love to hear her speak, yet well I know
That music hath a far more pleasing sound;
I grant I never saw a goddess go;
My mistress, when she walks, treads on the ground:
And yet, by heaven, I think my love as rare
As any she belied with false compare.

Sonnet CXXX

Call me but love, and I'll be new baptis'd.

Romeo and Juliet

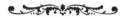

Where hast thou been, my heart?

Antony and Cleopatra

Fair one, all goodness that consists in beauty.

Pericles

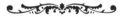

Soft, I will go along;
And if you leave me so, you do me wrong.

Romeo and Juliet

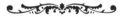

So holy and perfect is my love,
And I in such a poverty of grace,
That I shall think it a most plenteous crop
To glean the broken ears after the man
That the main harvest reaps; loose now and then
A scattered smile, and that I'll live upon.

As You Like It

Wouldst thou then counsel me to fall in love?

The Two Gentlemen of Verona

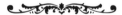

Now my lord, what say you to my suit?

Romeo and Juliet

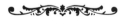

The fairest that I have look'd upon.

Cymbeline

You must lay down the treasures of your body.

Measure for Measure

The sweetest flower of all the field.

Romeo and Juliet

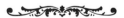

. . . a shop of all the qualities that man
Loves woman for.

Cymbeline

Where is my wit? I know not what I speak.

Troilus and Cressida

You are a lover, borrow Cupid's wings
And soar with them above a common bound.

Romeo and Juliet

I would I were invisible, to catch the strong fellow by the leg.

As You Like It

'Tis [your] breathing that
Perfumes the chamber thus.

Cymbeline

Dumb jewels often in their silent kind,
More than quick words, do move a woman's mind.

The Two Gentlemen of Verona

Here pleasures court mine eyes.

Pericles

The air . . . for vacancy,
Had gone to gaze on [you]
And made a gap in nature.

All's Well That Ends Well

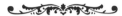

You have a nimble wit.

As You Like It

Most radiant, exquisite, and unmatchable beauty!

Twelfth Night

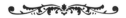

Heaven and earth . . . do meet in thee at once.

Romeo and Juliet

Plainly conceive, I love you.

Measure for Measure

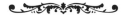

[Thy] virtue and . . . general graces speak
That which none else can utter.

Antony and Cleopatra

Mcthinks I feel this youth's perfections
With an invisible and subtle stealth
To creep in at mine eyes.

Twelfth Night

Black men are pearls in beauteous ladies eyes.

The Two Gentlemen of Verona

What a paragon!

Pericles

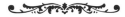

Good marrow, fairest.

Cymbeline

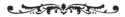

They that dally nicely with words may quickly make them wanton.

Twelfth Night

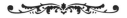

Look where thy love comes; yonder is thy dear.

A Midsummer Night's Dream

. . . Not so fair . . . as well-favored.

The Two Gentlemen of Verona

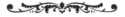

Jove, Jove! This shepherd's passion
Is much upon my fashion.

As You Like It

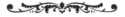

You do usurp yourself: for what is yours to bestow is
not yours to reserve.

Twelfth Night

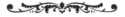

One of the noblest note.

Cymbeline

My ears have not yet drunk a hundred words
Of thy tongue's uttering, yet I know the sound.

Romeo and Juliet

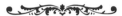

Look how fresh she looks!

Pericles

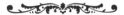

I conclusion, I stand affected . . .

The Two Gentlemen of Verona

'Tis beauty truly blent, whose red and white
nature's own sweet and cunning hand laid on.

Twelfth Night

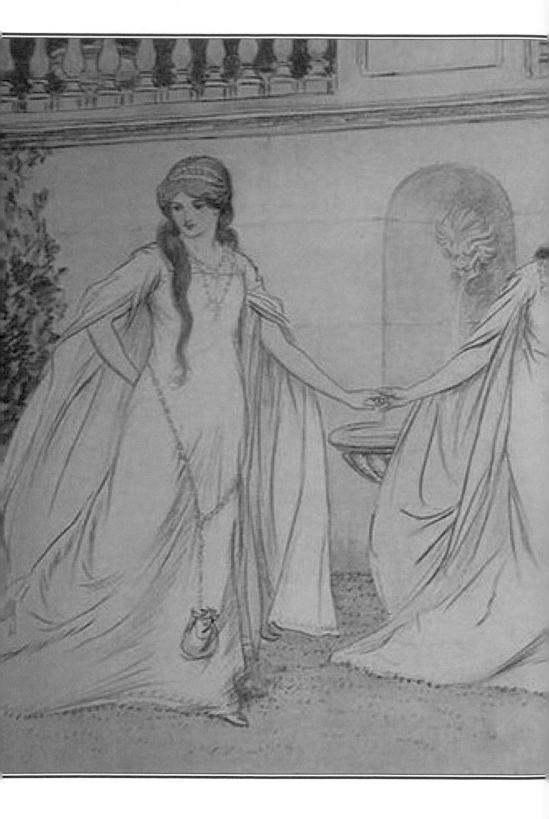

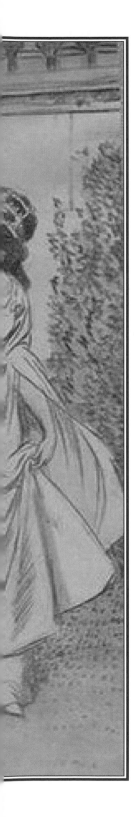

Love's Seductions

Men's eyes were made to look, and let them gaze.

Romeo and Juliet

Out of my sight! thou dost infect my eyes.
Thine eyes, sweet lady, have infected mine.

Richard III

They have the plague, and caught it of your eyes.

Love's Labour's Lost

I think I shall have something to do with you.

Pericles

Hearing thy mildness prais'd in every town,
Thy virtues spoke of, and thy beauty sounded,
Yet not so deeply as to thee belongs,
Myself am mov'd to woo thee for my wife.

The Taming of the Shrew

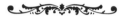

It is not politic in the commonwealth of nature to
preserve virginity.

All's Well That Ends Well

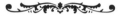

Give me swift transportation to those field
Where I may wallow in the lily beds.

Troilus and Cressida

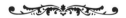

Trust me, sweet.

A Midsummer Night's Dream

Please you, draw me near.

The Tempest

Come woo me, woo me; for I am in a holiday humor and like to consent.

As You Like It

Here's much to do with hate, but more with love.

Romeo and Juliet

Come, sit on me.

The Taming of the Shrew

If I could win a lady at leap-frog, or by vaulting into
my saddle with my armour on my back, under the
correction of bragging be it spoken. I should quickly
leap into a wife.
Or if I might buffet for my love, or bound my horse
for her favours, I could lay on like a butcher and sit
like a jack-an-apes, never off. But, before God, Kate, I
cannot look greenly nor gasp out my eloquence, nor
I have no cunning in protestation; only downright
oaths, which I never use till urged, nor never break
for urging. If thou canst love a fellow of this temper,
Kate, whose face is not worth sun-burning, that never
looks in his glass for love of any thing he sees there,
let thine eye be thy cook. I speak to thee plain soldier:
If thou canst love me for this, take me: if not, to say
to thee that I shall die, is true; but for thy love, by the
Lord, no; yet I love thee too.

Henry V

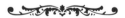

Such a passion doth embrace my bosom.

Troilus and Cressida

If thou lov'st me then,
Steal forth thy father's house tomorrow night;
And in the wood, a league without the town. . .
There will I stay for thee.

A Midsummer Night's Dream

What cheer?

The Tempest

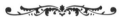

All hail the richest beauties on the earth!

Love's Labour's Lost

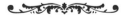

Pray you, come hither awhile.

Pericles

My love can give no place, bide no delay.

Twelfth Night

In delay we waste our lights in vain.

Romeo and Juliet

My manly eyes did scorn an humble tear;
And what these sorrows could not thence exhale,
Thy beauty hath, and made them blind with weeping.
I never sued to friend nor enemy;
My tongue could never learn sweet smoothing word;
But now thy beauty is proposed my fee,
My proud heart sues, and prompts my tongue to speak.

Richard III

I do beseech you pardon me:
'Twas not my purpose thus to beg a kiss.

Troilus and Cressida

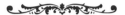

Love, lend me wings to make my purpose swift
As thou hast lent me wit to plot this drift.

The Two Gentlemen of Verona

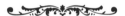

O, come hither.

Pericles

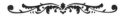

Hast thou not dropped from heaven?

The Tempest

43

Lady, give me your hand, and, as we walk,
To our own selves bend we our needful talk.

Troilus and Cressida

❧

Are you meditating on virginity?

All's Well That Ends Well

❧

O, I am yours, and all that I possess.

Love's Labour's Lost

❧

Then bid me kill myself, and I will do it.

Richard III

There lies more peril in thine eye
Than twenty . . . swords. Look thou but sweet
And I am proof against their enmity.

Romeo and Juliet

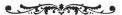

Night hath been too brief.

Troilus and Cressida

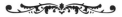

Why lament you pretty one?

Pericles

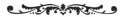

I do beseech you—
Chiefly that I might set it in my prayers—
What is your name?

The Tempest

Run through fire I will for thy sweet sake!

A Midsummer Night's Dream

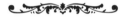

Give me some music—music, moody food
Of us that trade in love.

Antony and Cleopatra

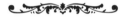

Your heart's desires be with you.

As You Like It

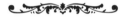

Come, young one, I like the manner of your garments
well.

Pericles

I will show you a chamber with a bed, which bed,
because it shall not speak of your pretty encounter,
press it to death!

Troilus and Cressida

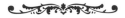

My prime request,
Which I do last pronounce, is, O you wonder!
If you be maid or no?

The Tempest

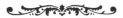

By heaven, that thou art fair, is most infallible; true,
that thou art beauteous; truth itself, that thou art
lovely. More fairer than fair, beautiful than beauteous,
truer than truth itself, have commiseration on thy
heroical vassal!

Love's Labour's Lost

Come hither, boy, If ever thou shalt love,
In the sweet pangs of it remember me:
For such as I am, all true lovers are,
Unstaid and skittish in all motions else,
Save in the constant image of the creature
That is belov'd. How dost thou like this tune?

Twelfth Night

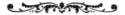

Will you not go the way of woman-kind?

Pericles

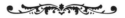

I prithee now, to bed.

Troilus and Cressida

Vouchsafe me for my meed but one fair look;
A smaller boon than this I cannot beg,
And less than this I am sure you cannot give.

The Two Gentlemen of Verona

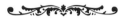

How now, you wanton calf!
Art thou my calf?

The Winter's Tale

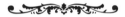

I long
To hear the story of your life, which must
Take the ear strongly.

The Tempest

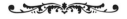

You have fortunes coming upon you.

Pericles

Let me have audience for a word or two.

As You Like It

Come young waverer, come, go with me.

Romeo and Juliet

White-handed mistress, one sweet word with you.

Love's Labour's Lost

Thou hast metamorphos'd me;
Made me neglect my studies, lose my time,
Here, wear this jewel for me, 'tis my picture:
Refuse it not, it hath no tongue to vex you:
And I beseech you come again tomorrow.

Twelfth Night

I'll look to like if looking liking move.

Romeo and Juliet

⁂

War with good counsel, set the world at naught;
Made wit with musing weak, heart sick with thought.

The Two Gentlemen of Verona

⁂

I desire with all my heart; and I hope it is no
dishonest desire, to desire to be a woman of the
world.

As You Like It

⁂

Henceforth my wooing mind shall be express'd
In russet yeas and honest kersey noes:
And, to begin: Wench,—so God help me, law—
My love to thee is sound, sans crack or flaw.

Love's Labour's Lost

I am too bold.

Romeo and Juliet

. . . I held this hand, whose touch
. . . would force the feeler's soul
To th'oath of loyalty.

Cymbeline

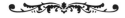

Where dwell you pretty youth?

As You Like It

Sweet lady, entertain . . .

The Two Gentlemen of Verona

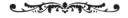

I'll be thine, my fair.

The Winter's Tale

If a virgin,
And your affection not gone forth, I'll make you
The queen of Naples.

The Tempest

I prithee, pretty youth, let me be better acquainted
with thee.

As You Like It

If it please you, so; if not, why, so.

The Two Gentlemen of Verona

There is no tongue that moves, none,
none i' th' world,
So soon as yours, could win me.

The Winter's Tale

O, sweetest, fairest lily.

Cymbeline

❦

I sit possible, that on so little acquaintance you should like? That but seeing, you should love? And loving woo? And wooing, should grant?

As You Like It

❦

Madam and mistress, a thousand good-morrows.

The Two Gentlemen of Verona

❦

I have an eye of you. If you love me, hold not off.

Hamlet

You'd wanton with us,
If we would have you.

The Winter's Tale

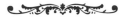

Why do you look on me?

As You Like It

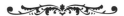

If the gentle spirit of moving words
Can no way change you to a milder form,
I'll woo you like a soldier, at arms end,
And love you 'gainst the nature of love:
force ye.

The Two Gentlemen of Verona

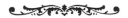

Still I swear I love you.

Cymbeline

My errand is to you, fair youth.

As You Like It

That man hath a tongue, I say is no man,
If with his tongue he cannot win a woman.

The Two Gentlemen of Verona

Let us talk in good earnest: Is it possible, on such a
sudden, you should fall into so strong a liking?

As You Like It

My desires
Run not before mine honor, nor my lusts
Burn hotter than my faith.

The Winter's Tale

Maids in modesty, say "no" to that
Which they would have the profferer construe "ay."

The Two Gentlemen of Verona

How now, boy?

The Winter's Tale

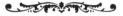

What should a man do but be merry?

Hamlet

I am not furnished like a beggar, therefore to beg will
not become me. My way is to conjure you.

As You Like It

I love this lady too-too much.

The Two Gentlemen of Verona

You'll kiss me hard, and speak to me as if I were a baby still.

The Winter's Tale

Upon her landing, Antony sent to her,
Invited her to supper; she replied,
I would be better he became her guest;
Which she entreated: our courteous Antony
Whom ne'er the word of "No" woman heard speak,
Being barber'd ten time o'er, goes to the feast,
And, for his ordinary, pays his heart
For what his eyes eat only.

Antony and Cleopatra

What is this? Sport?

The Winter's Tale

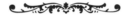

This music crept by me upon the waters,
Allaying both their fury and my passion
With its sweet air.

The Tempest

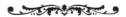

From henceforth I will . . . devise sports. Let me see,
what think you of falling in love?

As You Like It

Do not you chide, I have a thing for you.

Othello

We two will walk.

The Winter's Tale

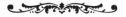

The object and pleasure of mine eye.

A Midsummer Night's Dream

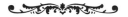

Follow mc girls.

The Winter's Tale

I set thee in a shower of gold and hail
Rich pearls upon thee.

Antony and Cleopatra

Wish me partaker in thy happiness
When thou dost meet good hap.

The Two Gentlemen of Verona

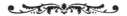

Come, stand not amazed . . . but go along
with me.

Othello

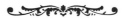

Heaven is here where you live.

Romeo and Juliet

If you will be married tomorrow, you shall.

As You Like It

What made me love thee?
Honey, you shall be well desired.

Othello

Ask me no reason why I love you

The Merry Wives of Windsor

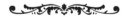

Your ladyship is nearer to heaven than when I saw you
last.

Hamlet

Your praises are too large.

The Winter's Tale

The hand that hath made you fair hath made
you good.

Love's Labour's Lost

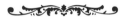

To plead for love deserves more fee than hate.

The Two Gentlemen of Verona

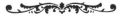

You're a fair creature.

All's Well That Ends Well

I thank thee for that jest.

The Tempest

Touch but my lips with those fair lips of thine,—
Though mine be not so fair, yet they are red,—
The kiss shall be thine own as well as mine:
What seest thou on the ground? Hold up
thy head:
Look in mine eyeballs, there thy beauty lies;
Then why not lips on lips, since eyes in eyes?

Venus and Adonis

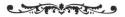

What is your name?

Twelfth Night

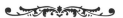

I am angling now,
Though you perceive me not how I give line.

The Winter's Tale

I life would wish, and that I might
Waste it for you like taper-light.

Pericles

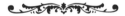

Some love of yours hast writ to you in rhyme.

The Two Gentlemen of Verona

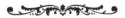

How do you, pretty lady?

Hamlet

I'll follow thee, and make a heaven of hell.

A Midsummer Night's Dream

You are not young, no more am I; go to, then, there's sympathy. You are merry, so am I; ha, ha, then, there's more sympathy. You love sack, and so do I; would you desire better sympathy?

The Merry Wives of Windsor

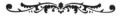

I am at war 'twixt will and will not.

Measure for Measure

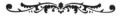

Consent . . . that we may enjoy each other.

As You Like It

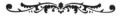

I desire better acquaintance.

Twelfth Night

I pray . . . come a little nearer this ways.

The Merry Wives of Windsor

Thy love ne'er alter till thy sweet life end!

A Midsummer Night's Dream

And when great treasure is the meed proposed,
Though death be adjunct, there's no death supposed.

The Rape of Lucrece

I love thee; help me away. Let me creep
in there.

The Merry Wives of Windsor

Love, lend me wings to make my purpose swift
As thou hast lent me wit to plot this drift.

The Two Gentleman of Verona

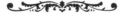

Come, you'll play with me, sir?

Antony and Cleopatra

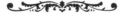

Assure thyself there is no love-broker in the world can
more prevail in man's commendation with woman
than report of valor.

Twelfth Night

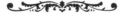

[Your] fingers are long, small, white as milk.

Pericles

What would you with me?

The Merry Wives of Windsor

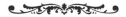

I see, sir, you are eaten up with passion.

Othello

She was never yet that ever knew
Love got so sweet as when desire did sue.

Troilus and Cressida

Fit thy consent to my sharp appetite.

Measure for Measure

I am your spaniel . . .
The more you beat me, I will fawn on you.
Use me but as your spaniel, spurn me, strike me,
Neglect me, lose me; only give me leave,
Unworthy as I am, to follow you.

A Midsummer Night's Dream

Come, give us a taste of your quality.

Hamlet

Where did you learn this goodly speech?

The Taming of the Shrew

[Thou art in love if]
. . . first you have learned . . . to wreathe your arms like
a malcontent; to relish a love song, like a robin-breast;
to walk alone, like one that had the pestilence; to sigh,
like a schoolboy that had lost his ABC; to weep, like a
young wench that had buried her grandma; to fast, like
on that takes diet; to watch, like on that fears robbing;
to speak puling like a beggar at Hollowmas.

The Two Gentlemen of Verona

Nay, do not pause; for I did kill King Henry,
But 'twas thy beauty that provoked me.
Nay, now dispatch; 'twas I that stabb'd young Edward,
But 'twas thy heavenly face that set me on.

Richard III

I love you better . . . not for because
Your brows are blacker, yet black brows, they say,
Become some women best, so that there be not
Too much hair there, but in a semicircle,
Or half-moon made with a pen.

The Winter's Tale

[You are] a goodly creature.

Pericles

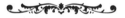

Send me a cool rut-time, Jove.

The Merry Wives of Windsor

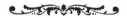

Let no man mock me,
For I will kiss.

The Winter's Tale

Vouchsafe, thou wonder, to alight thy steed
And rein his proud head to the saddle-bow;
If thou wilt deign this favor, for thy meed
A thousand honey secrets shalt thou know:
Here come and sit, where never serpent hisses;
And being set, I'll smother thee with kisses:

Venus and Adonis

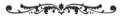

Come! Come buy!
Buy, lads, or else your lasses cry.

The Winter's Tale

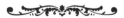

O flatter me; for love delights in praises.

The Two Gentlemen of Verona

How now, good woman, how dost thou?

The Merry Wives of Windsor

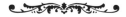

O mistress mine where are you roaming?
O stay and hear your true love's coming,
   That can sing both high and low.
   Trip no further, pretty sweeting:
   Journeys end in lovers meeting,
   Every wise man's son doth know.

   What is love? 'Tis not hereafter,
   Present mirth hath present laughter:
   What's to come is still unsure.
   In delay there lies no plenty,
   Then come kiss me, sweet and twenty:
   Youth's a stuff will not endure.

Twelfth Night

Come up to my chamber.

The Merry Wives of Windsor

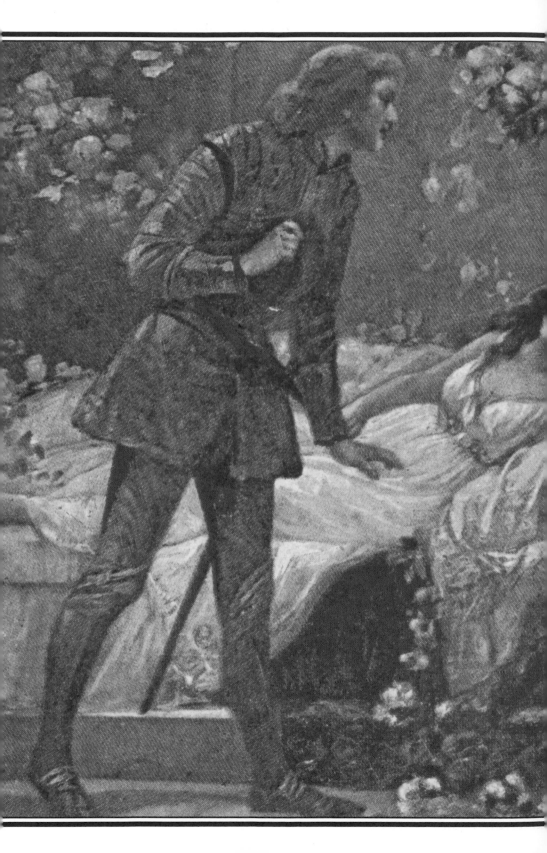

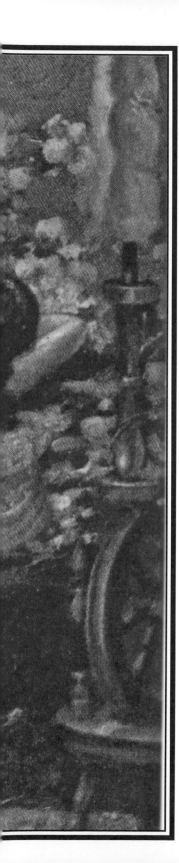

Love
in
Action

(Acts of Love)

Quench the fire, the room has grown too hot.

Romeo and Juliet

I come to whet your gentle thoughts.

Twelfth Night

Hush, and be mute, or else our spell is marr'd.

The Tempest

You have been hotly called for.

Othello

That's affair thought to lie between maid's legs.

Hamlet

You smile and mock me, as if I meant naughtily.

Troilus and Cressida

. . . give me the potions and the motions.

The Merry Wives of Windsor

If love be rough with you, be rough with love.

Romeo and Juliet

Come, bring me to some private place; come, come.

Pericles

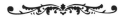

Mistress, know yourself. Down on your knees
And thank heaven, fasting, for a good
man's love.

As You Like It

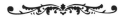

Thus have I had thee, as a dream doth flatter,
In sleep a king, but waking no such matter.

Sonnet LXXXVII

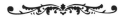

It is common for the younger sort
To lack discretion.

Hamlet

Madam, undress you and come now to bed.

The Taming of the Shrew

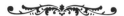

I will be correspondent to command.

The Tempest

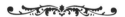

Though the chameleon Love can feed on the air, I am one that am nourished by my vituals; and would fain have meat.

The Two Gentlemen of Verona

Thank me no thinkings nor proud me no prouds,
But fettle your fine joints.

Romeo and Juliet

They say all lovers swear more performance than they
are able.

Troilus and Cressida

His hand, that yet remains upon her breast,—
Rude ram, to batter such an ivory wall!—
May feel her heart-poor citizen!—distress'd,
Wounding itself to death, rise up and fall,
Beating her bulk, that his hand shakes withal.
This moves in him more rage and lesser pity,
To make the breach and enter this sweet city.

The Rape of Lucrece

Flow, flow,
You heavenly blessings.

Cymbeline

Now comes the wanton blood up in your cheeks.
They'll be in scarlet straight.

Romeo and Juliet

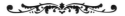

Now, the hot-blooded gods assist me!

The Merry Wives of Windsor

My naked weapon is out.

Romeo and Juliet

You are keen, my lord, you are keen.

Hamlet

I'll do the service of a younger man
In all your business and necessities.

As You Like It

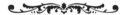

If love be blind, love cannot hit the mark.

Romeo and Juliet

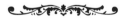

Go, play, boy, play.

The Winter's Tale

Heaven prosper our sport!

The Merry Wives of Windsor

What shall be out sport then?

As You Like It

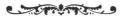

I should kill thee with much cherishing.

Romeo and Juliet

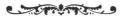

Eat nothing but doves, love, and that breed hot blood, and hot blood begets hot thoughts, and hot thoughts beget hot deeds, and hot deeds is love.

Troilus and Cressida

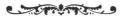

Raise up the organs of fantasy.

The Merry Wives of Windsor

Draw thy tool.

Romeo and Juliet

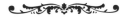

O excellent motion! O exceeding puppet!

The Two Gentlemen of Verona

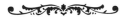

O God's lady dear,
Are you so hot?

Romeo and Juliet

Sweet lady, ho, ho!

Twelfth Night

I do not desire you to please me, I do desire you
to sing.

As You Like It

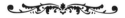

Now, tell me how long you would have, after you
have possessed?

As You Like It

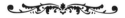

Against such lewdsters and their lechery
Those that betray them do no treachery.

The Merry Wives of Windsor

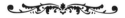

If this be magic, let it be an art
Lawful as eating.

The Winter's Tale

Let lips do what hands do.

Romeo and Juliet

❧

[Let's] embrace, kiss, protest, and, as it were, speak
the prologue of our comedy.

The Merry Wives of Windsor

❧

It would cost you a groaning to take off my edge.

Hamlet

❧

Look
I draw the sword myself, take it, and hit
The innocent mansion of my love, my heart:
Fear not, 'tis empty of all things, but grief:

Cymbeline

O, contain yourself:
Your passion draws ears hither.

Troilus and Cressida

What is your pleasure?

Othello

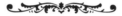

Prick love for pricking and you beat love down.

Romeo and Juliet

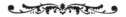

Though I look old, yet I am strong and lusty.

As You Like It

There's not a minute of your lives should stretch
Without some pleasure now. What sport tonight?

Antony and Cleopatra

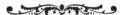

Not so hot, good sir.

The Winter's Tale

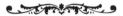

Thou art a piece of virtue.

Pericles

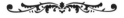

Thou mak'st me merry; I am full of pleasure.
Let us be jocund.

The Tempest

Other women cloy
The appetites they feed, but [you] make hungry
Where most you satisfy.

Antony and Cleopatra

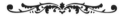

Quite athwart goes all decorum.

Measure for Measure

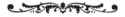

Thou hast amaz'd me.

Romeo and Juliet

Some rise by sin, and some by virtue fall.

Love's Labour's Lost

We should be woo'd and were not made to woo.

A Midsummer Night's Dream

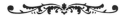

Methinks it is very sultry and hot for my complexion.

Hamlet

Young gentleman, your spirits are too bold for your years.

As You Like it

Thou hast been godlike perfect.

Pericles

With everything that pretty is, my lady sweet, arise;
Arise, arise!

Cymbeline

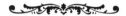

Be not afraid good youth, I will not have you.
And yet when wit and youth has come to harvest,
Your wife is like to reap a proper man.

Twelfth Night

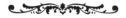

Why, is not this better now than groaning
for love?

Romeo and Juliet

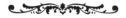

How now, friend Eros?

Antony and Cleopatra

Young sir, your reputation shall not . . . be misprized.

As You Like It

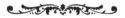

He burns with bashful shame; she with her tears
Doth quench the maiden burning of his cheeks;
    Then with her windy sighs and golden hairs
    To fan and blow them dry again she seeks:
    He saith she is immodest, blames her miss;
    What follows more she murders with a kiss.

Venus and Adonis

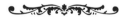

What a man are you?

Romeo and Juliet

What angel wakes me from my flowery bed?

A Midsummer Night's Dream

Give it me, it's mine.
Sweet ornament, that decks a thing divine!

The Two Gentlemen of Verona

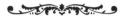

Here
My bluest veins to kiss.

Antony and Cleopatra

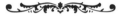

Now art thou sociable.

Romeo and Juliet

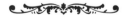

Let us withdraw together,
And we may soon our satisfaction have.

Measure for Measure

What art thou that usurp'st this time of night?

Hamlet

I dedicate myself to your sweet pleasure.

Cymbeline

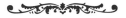

Fair maid, send forth thine eye.

All's Well That Ends Well

You are a saucy boy.

Romeo and Juliet

Oh, fear me not.

Hamlet

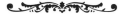

Where souls do couch on flowers we'll hand
in hand
And with your sprightly port make ghosts gaze.

Antony and Cleopatra

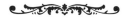

[Thy] love-suit hath been to me
As fearful as a siege.

Cymbeline

Soft, methinks I scent the morning air.

Hamlet

'Tis known I am a pretty piece of flesh.

Romeo and Juliet

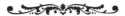

[You] put mettle in restrained means.

Love's Labour's Lost

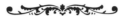

How bravely thou become'st thy bed!

Cymbeline

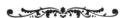

I am the very pink of courtesy.

Romeo and Juliet

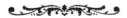

Am I the Man yet?

As You Like It

I'll blush you thanks.

The Winter's Tale

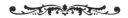

I'll make a journey twice as far, t'enjoy
A second night of such sweet shortness.

Cymbeline

Yet hold off. Women are angels, wooing:
Things won are done; joy's soul lies in
the doing.

Troilus and Cressida

Spend that kiss
Which is my heaven to have.

Antony and Cleopatra

We will begin these rites,
As we do trust they'll end, in true delights.

As You Like It

Strike me . . .
Give me a gash, put me to present pain,
Lest this great sea of joys rushing upon me
O'er bear the shores of my mortality,
And drown me with their sweetness.

Pericles

When good will is showed, though't come too short,
The actor may plead pardon.

Antony and Cleopatra

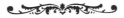

Come, come, wrestle with thy affections.

As You Like It

What early tongue so sweet saluteth me?

Romeo and Juliet

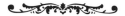

O come, let us remove.

As You Like It

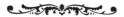

Mine, and most of our fortunes tonight, shall be drunk to bed.

Antony and Cleopatra

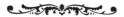

I search it with a sovereign kiss.

The Two Gentlemen of Verona

Give me your hand . . .
Then learn this of me. To have is to have.

As You Like It

I come, my queen.

Antony and Cleopatra

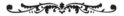

Here comes a spirit.

The Tempest

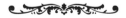

Not so fast: soft! Soft!

Twelfth Night

That I might touch!
But kiss! One kiss.

Cymbeline

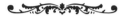

Love give me strength.

Romeo and Juliet

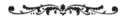

Come, my queen!
Last night you did desire it.

Antony and Cleopatra

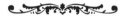

Let none disturb us.

Pericles

I would kiss before I spoke.

As You Like It

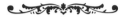

Wilt thou go to bed?

Twelfth Night

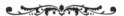

Why, how know you that I am in love?

The Two Gentlemen of Verona

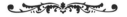

Come, let's have another gaudy night.

Antony and Cleopatra

Very good, well kissed and excellent courtesy; 'tis so indeed!

Othello

What passion hangs these weights upon my tongue?

As You Like It

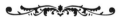

You have the honey.

Troilus and Cressida

Thou cut'st my head off with a golden axe
And smilest upon the stroke that murders me.

Romeo and Juliet

Thy tongue, thy face, thy limbs, actions, and spirit
Do give thee five-fold blazon.

Twelfth Night

You shall be yet far fairer than you are.

Antony and Cleopatra

O how I love thee! How I dote on thee!

A Midsummer Night's Dream

I am a maid,
. . . that ne'er before invited eyes,
but have been gazed on like a comet.

Pericles

By my life,
. . . I kissed it, give me present hunger
To feed again, though full.

Cymbeline

What great ones do, the less with prattle of.

Twelfth Night

Well said! Thou lookst cheerly, and I'll be with you
quickly.

As You Like it

Come sit thee down upon this flowery bed,
While I thy amiable cheeks do coy,
And stick musk-roses in thy sleek smooth head,
And kiss thy fair large ears, my gentle joy.

A Midsummer Night's Dream

Give me your hand sir.

Twelfth Night

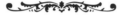

Give me a kiss.
Even this repays it.

Antony and Cleopatra

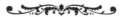

Afore God I am so vexed that every part about me
quivers.

Romeo and Juliet

Let me my service tender on your lips.

Cymbeline

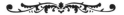

To bed? Ay, sweetheart, and I'll come to thee.

Twelfth Night

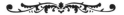

Thy lips are warm.

Romeo and Juliet

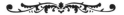

Prised be the gods for thy foulness; sluttishness may come hereafter. But be that as it may be, I will marry thee.

As You Like It

That were to blow at fire in hope to quench it.

Pericles

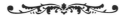

I would I were thy bird.

Romeo and Juliet

O let me kiss
This princess of pure white, this seal of bliss.

A Midsummer Night's Dream

And now this lustful lord leap'd from his bed,
Throwing his mantle rudely o'er his arm;
Is madly toss'd between desire and dread;
Th' one sweetly flatters, th' other feareth harm;
But honest fear, bewitch'd with lust's foul charm,
Doth too too oft betake him to retire,
Beaten away by brain-sick rude desire.

The Rape of Lucrece

O spirit of love, how quick and fresh art thou!

Twelfth Night

Nay, come, your hands and lips must seal it too.

Pericles

I will lie with thee tonight.

Romeo and Juliet

For, lo, his passion, but an art of craft,
Even there resolved my reason into tears;
There my white stole of chastity I daff'd,
Shook off my sober guards and civil fears;
Appear to him, as he to me appears,
All melting; though our drops this difference bore,
His poison'd me, and mine did him restore.

A Lover's Complaint

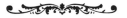

Come on, my queen,
There's sap in't yet!

Antony and Cleopatra

My wit faints.

Romeo and Juliet

My love is strengthen'd, though more weak in seeming;
I love not less, though less the show appear.

Sonnet CII

Have I caught thee, my heavenly jewel?

The Merry Wives of Windsor

I'll take that winter from your lips, fair lady.

Troilus and Cressida

Come, give me your flowers.

Pericles

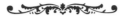

Yield up thy body to my will.

Measure for Measure

Hymen's lamps shall light thee.

The Tempest

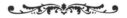

If I profane with my unworthiest hand
This holy shrine, the gentle sin is this:
My lips two blushing pilgrims, ready stand
To smooth that rough touch with a tender kiss.

Romeo and Juliet

It is legs and thighs. Let me see thee caper. Ha,
higher!

Twelfth Night

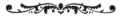

How achiev'd you these endowments . . . ?

Pericles

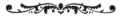

My love thou art, my love I think!

A Midsummer Night's Dream

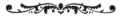

On touching of [your] lips I may melt.

Pericles

I will kiss thy lips.

Romeo and Juliet

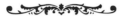

I come to answer thy best pleasure.

The Tempest

Sleep for a week; for the next night. . .you shall rest but little!

Romeo and Juliet

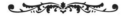

Performance shall follow.

Pericles

Setting the attraction of my good parts aside, I have
no other charms.

The Merry Wives of Windsor

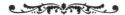

Doff thy name,
And for thy name, which is no part of thee,
Take all myself.

Romeo and Juliet

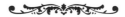

Sleep thou, and I will wind thee in my arms.

A Midsummer Night's Dream

Lend thy hand, and pluck my magic garment from me.

The Tempest

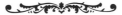

O wilt thou leave me so unsatisfied?

Romeo and Juliet

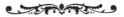

Pleasure and action make the hours seem short.

Othello

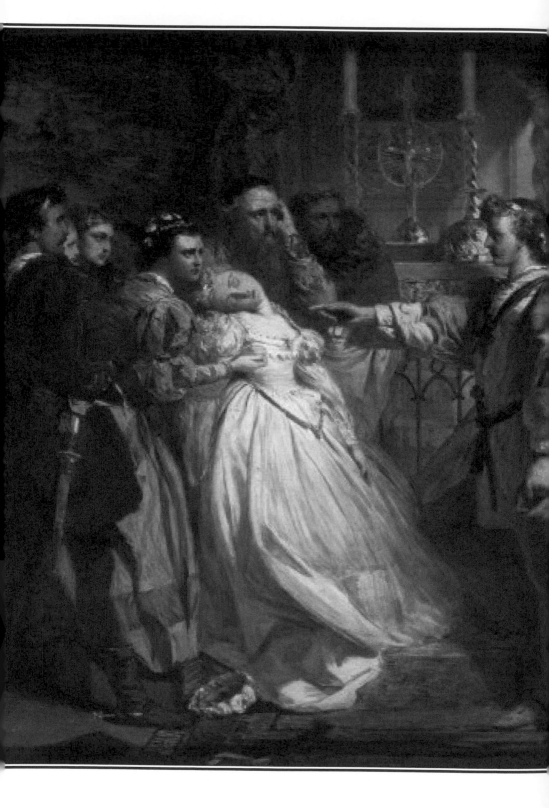

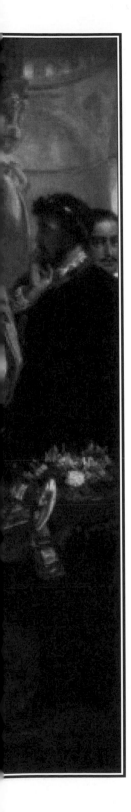

Inconstant Love

O swear not by the moon, th' inconstant moon,
That monthly changes in her circled orb,
Lest that thy love prove likewise variable.

Romeo and Juliet

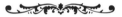

This is the monstrosity in love, lady: that the will is
infinite, and the execution confined: that the desire is
boundless, and the act a slave to limit.

Troilus and Cressida

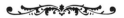

Pray, chuck, come hither.

Othello

How now, wholesome iniquity?

Pericles

How now fair maid?

Measure for Measure

———❧———

Look how well my garments sit upon me.

The Tempest

———❧———

Blind is his love, and best befits the dark.

Romeo and Juliet

———❧———

Let thy song be love: this love will undo us all.

Troilus and Cressida

———❧———

Price you yourselves: what buys your company?

Love's Labour's Lost

Happily, you something know.

Measure for Measure

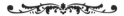

To take is not to give.

Richard III

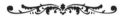

'Twas never merry world
Since lowly feigning was call'd compliment.

Twelfth Night

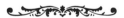

O, these men, these men!

Othello

Most dangerous
Is that temptation that doth goad us on
To sin in loving virtue.

Measure for Measure

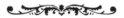

You are well favor'd, and your looks forshow
You have a gentle heart.

Pericles

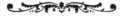

Now, by the world, it is a lusty wench.

The Taming of the Shrew

I flam'd amazement.

The Tempest

126

You rise to play, and go to bed to work.

Othello

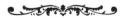

Is love a tender thing? It is too rough
Too rude, too boisterous, and it pricks like thorn.

Romeo and Juliet

We two, that with so many thousand sighs
Did buy each other . . .

Troilus and Cressida

Love bade me swear, and love bids me foreswear.

The Two Gentlemen of Verona

"Lucrece," quoth he, "this night I must enjoy thee:
If thou deny, then force must work my way,
For in thy bed I purpose to destroy thee:
That done, some worthless slave of thine I'll slay,
To kill thine honour with thy life's decay;
And in thy dead arms do I mean to place him,
Swearing I slew him, seeing thee embrace him."

The Rape of Lucrece

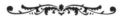

My actions are as noble as my thoughts.

Pericles

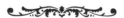

Might there not be a charity in sin?

Measure for Measure

Take a good heart, and counterfeit to be
a man.

As You Like It

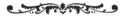

Beauty stirs up the lewdly inclin'd.

Pericles

Our indiscretion sometime serves us well.

Hamlet

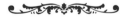

The bawdy hand of the dial is now upon the prick of
noon.

Romeo and Juliet

Such hazard now must doting Tarquin make,
Pawning his honour to obtain his lust;
And for himself himself be must forsake:
Then where is truth, if there be no self-trust?
When shall he think to find a stranger just,
When he himself himself confounds, betrays
To slanderous tongues and wretched hateful days?

The Rape of Lucrece

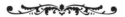

She belov'd knows naught that knows not this:
Men prize the thing ungain'd more than it is.

Troilus and Cressida

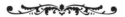

Have a shorter journey to your desires.

Othello

The mistress which I serve quickens what's dead
And makes my labours pleasures.

The Tempest

Come, the gods have done their part in you.

Pericles

Fate ordains [thou] should be a cuckold.

The Merry Wives of Windsor

Let it not gall your patience . . .
That I extend my manners; 'tis my breeding
That gives me this bold show of courtesy.

Othello

The error of our eyes directs our mind.

Troilus and Cressida

O serpent heart, hid with a flowering face.

Romeo and Juliet

You gods, that made me man, and sway in love,
That have inflam'd desire in my breast
To taste the fruit of yon celestial tree.

Pericles

I profess myself adorer, not friend.

Cymbeline

Thy thoughts I cleave to. What's thy pleasure.

The Tempest

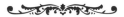

Now, pretty one, how long have you been at this trade?

Pericles

This unlooked for sport comes well.

Romeo and Juliet

My husband is thy friend; for his sake spare me:
Thyself art mighty; for thine own sake leave me.

The Rape of Lucrece

When nature fram'd this piece, she meant thee a good turn.

Pericles

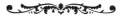

Fair youth, I would make thee believe I love.

As You Like It

You are wise,
Or else you love not; for to be wise and love
Exceeds man's might.

Troilus and Cressida

Precious creature.

The Tempest

. . . draw with spider's strings
Most ponderous and substantial things.

Love's Labour's Lost

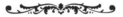

If thou swear'st . . .
Thou may prove false. At lovers' perjuries,
They say, Jove laughs.

Romeo and Juliet

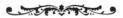

Who makes the fairest show means most deceit.

Pericles

What, are you married?

Measure for Measure

Believe, if you please, that I can do strange things.

As You Like it

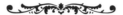

Dreamers often lie.

Romeo and Juliet

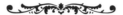

[You] will play with reason and discourse,
And well [you] can persuade.

Love's Labour's Lost

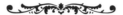

How much salt water thrown away in waste
To season love, that of it doth not taste.

Romeo and Juliet

My tricksy spirit!

The Tempest

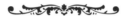

. . . saucy sweetness . . . coins heaven's image.

Measure for Measure

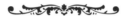

Pleasure's art can joy my spirit.

Pericles

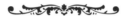

Surely, I think you have charms, la; yes in truth.

The Merry Wives of Windsor

[You are] a region in Giana, all gold and bounty.

Love's Labour's Lost

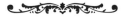

For further I could say "This man's untrue,"
And knew the patterns of his foul beguiling;
Heard where his plants in others' orchards grew,
Saw how deceits were gilded in his smiling;
Knew vows were ever brokers to defiling;
Thought characters and words merely but art,
And bastards of his foul adulterate heart.

A Lover's Complaint

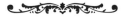

The tempter, or the tempted, who sins most, ha?

Measure for Measure

When the blood burns, how prodigal the soul
Lends the tongue vows.

Hamlet

Come every day to my cote, and woo me.

As You Like It

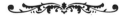

I pray come and crush a cup of wine.

Romeo and Juliet

Did I not dance with you in Brabant once?

Love's Labour's Lost

Why, lady, Love hath twenty pair of eyes.

The Two Gentlemen of Verona

So shall I live, supposing thou art true,
Like a deceived husband; so love's face
May still seem love to me, though alter'd new;
Thy looks with me, thy heart in other place:
For there can live no hatred in thine eye,
Therefore in that I cannot know thy change.
In many's looks the false heart's history
Is writ in moods and frowns and wrinkles strange,
But heaven in thy creation did decree
That in thy face sweet love should ever dwell;
Whate'er thy thoughts or thy heart's workings be,
Thy looks should nothing thence but sweetness tell.
How like Eve's apple doth thy beauty grow,
If thy sweet virtue answer not thy show!

Sonnet XCIII

When I break that oath, let me turn monster.

As You Like It

What sneaking fellow comes yonder?

Troilus and Cressida

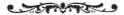

I like [your] money well.

The Merry Wives of Windsor

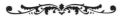

Tempt not a desperate man.

Romeo and Juliet

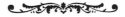

I do
Protest my ears were never better fed
With such delightful pleasing harmony.

Pericles

How came your eyes so bright?

A Midsummer Night's Dream

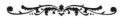

Let us be wary, let us hide our loves.

Othello

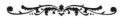

Beseech you, sir, be merry.

The Tempest

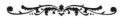

Love is not a hare that I do hunt.

As You Like It

Do you know a free man if you see him?

Troilus and Cressida

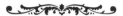

What revels are in hand?

Measure for Measure

Stand no more off,
But give thyself unto my sick desires.

All's Well That Ends Well

This is the third man that e'er I saw; the first
That e'er I sigh'd for.

The Tempest

Pretty virginity!

The Merry Wives of Windsor

Alas, what ignorant sin have I committed?

Othello

I do forgive thy robbery, gentle thief.

Sonnet XL

[You] are as all comforts are: most good, most good indeed.

Love's Labour's Lost

I [seek] the purchase of a glorious beauty.

Pericles

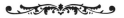

Full many a lady
I have ey'd with best regard, and many a time
Th'harmony of their tongues hath into bondage
Brought my too diligent ear; for several virtues
Have I lik'd several women; never any
With so full soul, but some defect in her
Did quarrel with the noblest grace she ow'd,
And put it in the foil: but you, O you,
So perfect and so peerless, are created
Of every creature's best.

The Tempest

Doth my simple feature content you?

As You Like It

Sweet, bid me hold my tongue,
For in this rapture I shall surely speak
The thing I shall repent.

Troilus and Cressida

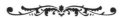

Here comes the trout that must be caught with
tickling.

Twelfth Night

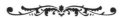

Ay me! I fell; and yet do question make
What I should do again for such a sake.

A Lover's Complaint

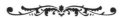

Thy will
By my performance shall be serv'd.

All's Well That Ends Well

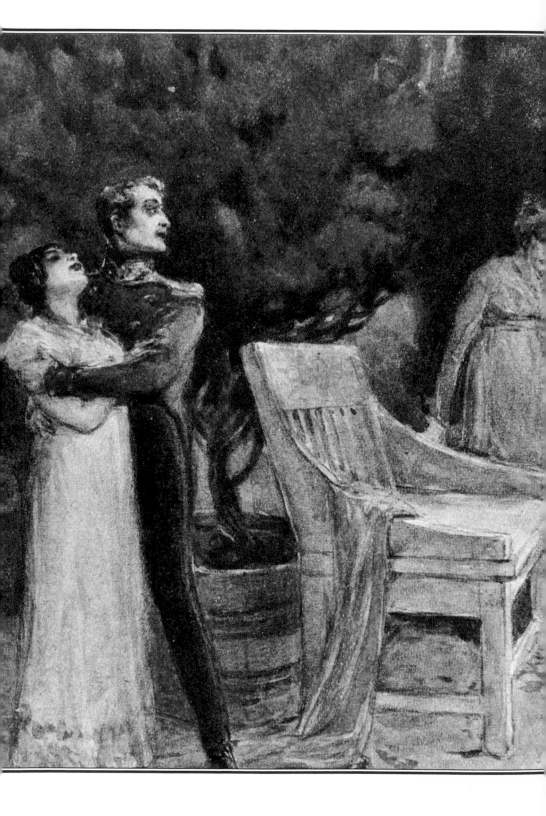

Love's Recriminations

Would you have me
False to my nature? Rather say I play
The man I am.

Coriolanus

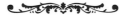

My only love sprung from my only hate.

Romeo and Juliet

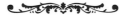

Dear, trouble not yourself; the morn is cold.

Troilus and Cressida

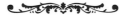

Sweet saint, for charity, be not so curst.

Richard III

[Thou art] too rough for me.

The Taming of the Shrew

⁂

I'll be wise hereafter,
And seek for grace. What a thrice-double ass
Was I, to take this drunkard for a good,
And worship this dull fool!

The Tempest

⁂

Fie, sirrah, a bawd, a wicked bawd!

Measure for Measure

⁂

I was mortally brought forth, and am
No other than I appear.

Pericles

Art thou afeard
To be the same in thine own act and valour
As thou art in desire? Wouldst thou have that
Which thou esteem'st the ornament of life,
And live a coward in thine own esteem,
Letting 'I dare not' wait upon 'I would,'
Like the poor cat i' the adage?

Macbeth

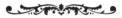

Here stand I, lady; dart thy skill at me;
Bruise me with scorn, confound me with a flout;
Thrust thy sharp wit quite through thy ignorance;
Cut me to pieces with thy keen conceit.

Love's Labour's Lost

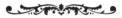

What says she, fair one? that the tongues of men
are full of deceits?

Henry V

O, that infected moisture of his eye,
O, that false fire which in his cheek so glow'd,
O, that forced thunder from his heart did fly,
O, that sad breath his spongy lungs bestow'd,
O, all that borrow'd motion seeming owed,
Would yet again betray the fore-betray'd,
And new pervert a reconciled maid!

A Lover's Complaint

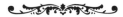

. . . I have lov'd you night and day
For many weary months.

Troilus and Cressida

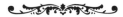

Thou driv'st me past the bounds
Of maiden's patience.

A Midsummer Night's Dream

Do you love, master? No?

The Tempest

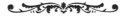

Why dost thou spit at me?
Never came poison from so sweet a place.

Richard III

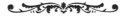

Arise fair sun and kill the envious moon
Who already sick and pale with grief
That thou her maid art far more fair than she.

Romeo and Juliet

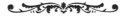

To make a sweet lady sad is a sour offence.

Troilus and Cressida

I will believe thee,
And make my senses credit thy relation
To points that seem impossible.

Pericles

Your wit's too hot, it speeds too fast, 'twill tire.

Love's Labour's Lost

Things base and vile, holding no quantity,
Love can transpose to form and dignity;
Love looks not with the eyes, but with the mind,
And therefore is wing'd Cupid painted blind;
Nor hath Love's mind of any judgment taste:
Wings, and no eyes, figure unheedy haste.
And therefore is Love said to be a child,
Because in choice he is so oft beguil'd.
As waggish boys, in game, themselves forswear,
So the boy Love is perjur'd everywhere.

A Midsummer Night's Dream

Words pay no debts.

Troilus and Cressida

Your tale, sir, would cure deafness.

The Tempest

She's not well married that lives married young.

Romeo and Juliet

I'll provide you a chain, and I'll do what I can to get you a pair of horns.

The Merry Wives of Windsor

But she hath lost a dearer thing than life,
And he hath won what he would lose again:
This forced league doth force a further strife;
This momentary joy breeds months of pain;
This hot desire converts to cold disdain:
Pure Chastity is rifled of her store,
And Lust, the thief, far poorer than before.

The Rape of Lucrece

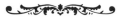

. . . Too fair. too wise, wisely too fair,
To merit bliss by making me despair.

Romeo and Juliet

. . . Thou art a man, and I
Have suffered like a girl.

Pericles

158

Go make thyself a nymph o' th' sea.

The Tempest

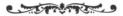

Now I do frown on thee with all my heart,
And if mine eyes can wound, now let them kill thee.

As You Like It

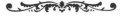

I will show more craft than love.

Troilus and Cressida

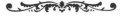

Wilt thou set thy foot o' my neck?

Twelfth Night

Let me remember thee what thou hast promis'd,
Which is not yet perform'd me.

The Tempest

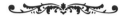

You men. You beasts!

Romeo and Juliet

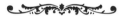

O that a lady, of one man refus'd,
Should of another therefore be abus'd.

A Midsummer Night's Dream

O beauty, where is thy faith?

Troilus and Cressida

Remember I have done thee worthy service;
Told thee no lies, made no mistakings, serv'd
Without grudge or grumblings.

The Tempest

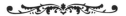

What win I, if I gain the thing I seek?
A dream, a breath, a froth of fleeting joy.
Who buys a minute's mirth to wail a week?
Or sells eternity to get a toy?
For one sweet grape who will the vine destroy?
Or what fond beggar, but to touch the crown,
Would with the sceptre straight be strucken down?

The Rape of Lucrece

Alas that love so gentle in his view
Should be so tyrannous and rough in proof.

Romeo and Juliet

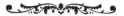

O heaven, you love me not!

Troilus and Cressida

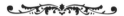

A fine volley of words, and quickly shot off.

The Two Gentlemen of Verona

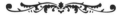

Sweet honey Greek, tempt me no more to folly.

Troilus and Cressida

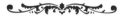

Look thou be true.

The Tempest

Good troth, you do me wrong, good sooth, you do,
In such disdainful manner me to woo.

A Midsummer Night's Dream

Rebuke me not for that which you provoke.

Love's Labour's Lost

I should have been more strange, I must confess,
But that thou overheard'st, ere I was ware,
My true-love passion.

Romeo and Juliet

You speak like one besotted on your sweet delights.

Troilus and Cressida

Sweet lord, you play me false.

The Tempest

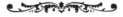

Many a good hanging prevents a bad marriage.

Twelfth Night

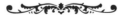

You are full of fair words.

Troilus and Cressida

Your bum is the greatest thing about you.

Measure for Measure

If ladies be but young and fair,
They have the gift to know it.

As You Like It

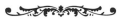

O teach me how I should forget to think.

Romeo and Juliet

The course of true love never did run smooth.

A Midsummer Night's Dream

You kiss by th' book.

Romeo and Juliet

Heaven make you better than your thoughts.

The Merry Wives of Windsor

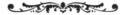

Did ever dragon keep so fair a cave?

Romeo and Juliet

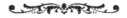

Why, this is very midsummer madness.

Twelfth Night

If you were men, as men you are in show,
You would not use a gentle lady so.

A Midsummer Night's Dream

Young men's love then lies
Not truly in their hearts but in their eyes.

Romeo and Juliet

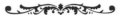

I care not for you.

Cymbeline

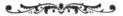

Fie, fie; how wayward is this foolish love,
That (like a testy babe) will scratch the nurse,
And presently all humbled kiss the rod!

The Two Gentlemen of Verona

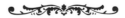

These are the forgeries of jealousy.

A Midsummer Night's Dream

Marry sir, sometimes [you] are a kind of Puritan.

Twelfth Night

I do not know . . . what I should think.

Hamlet

Beware my censure and keep your promise.

As You Like It

These times of woe afford no times to woo.

Romeo and Juliet

Is this the generation of love? Hot blood, hot thoughts, and hot deeds? Why, they are vipers. Is love a generation of vipers?

Troilus and Cressida

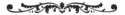

Sad, lady? I could be sad.

Twelfth Night

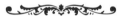

I love thee not, therefore pursue me not.

A Midsummer Night's Dream

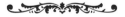

A man may be too confident.

The Merry Wives of Windsor

Your eye hath too much youth in 't.

The Winter's Tale

Go shake your ears.

Twelfth Night

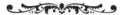

Well, go your way to her, for I see love hath made thee a tame snake.

As You Like It

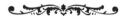

Thou canst not speak of that thou dost not feel.

Romeo and Juliet

Do I entice you? Do I speak you fair?
Or rather do I not in plainest truth
Tell you I do not, nor I cannot love you?

A Midsummer Night's Dream

Wherefore waste I time to counsel thee
That art a votery to fond desire.

The Two Gentlemen of Verona

Think you a little din can daunt mine ears?

The Taming of the Shrew

I have assail'd with musics, but [thou] vouchsafe no
notice.

Cymbeline

Talkest thou nothing but of ladies?

Twelfth Night

Pox of your love letters!

The Two Gentlemen of Verona

Teach not thy lips such scorn, for they were made
For kissing, lady, not for such contempt.
If thy revengeful heart cannot forgive,
Lo, here I lend thee this sharp-pointed sword;
Which if thou please to hide in this true bosom.
And let the soul forth that adoreth thee,
I lay it naked to the deadly stroke,
And humbly beg the death upon my knee.

Richard III

Be gone, solicit me no more.

The Two Gentlemen of Verona

Be gone, solicit me no more.

The worst fault you have is to be in love.

As You Like It

Might you dispense with your leisure, I would by and
by have some speech with you.

Measure for Measure

Oh why rebuke you him that loves you so?
Lay breath so bitter on your bitter foe.

A Midsummer Night's Dream

Think'st thou I am so shallow, so conceitless,
To be seduced by thy flattery,
That hast deceive'd so many with thy vows?

The Two Gentlemen of Verona

Deliver with more openness your answers
To my demands.

Cymbeline

I must tell you friendly in your ear,
Sell when you can, you are not for all markets.

As You Like It

Our love being yours, the error that love makes
Is likewise yours.

Love's Labour's Lost

Come, come do you think I do not know you by your excellent wit?

Much Ado About Nothing

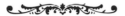

Pretty weathercock?

The Merry Wives of Windsor

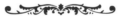

How now my headstrong; where have you been gadding?

Romeo and Juliet

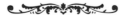

The wildest hath not such a heart as you.

A Midsummer Night's Dream

Come sir, I know what I know.

Measure for Measure

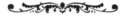

But it is certain I am loved of all ladies, only you excepted.

Much Ado About Nothing

Have I given any hard words of late?

Hamlet

Thy words are too precious to be cast away upon curs. Throw some of them at me; come, lame me with reasons.

As You Like It

How now, my love? Why is your cheek so pale?
How chance the roses there fade so fast?

A Midsummer Night's Dream

Entreat me how you can.

The Taming of the Shrew

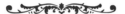

With an outstretch'd throat I'll tell the world aloud
What man thou art.

Love's Labour's Lost

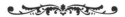

Nature cannot choose his origin.

Hamlet

I am so out of love with life.

Measure for Measure

A lover, or tyrant?

A Midsummer Night's Dream

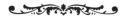

Thank God I am not a woman, to be touched with so many giddy offences as he hath generally taxed their whole sex with.

As You Like It

Bring forth men-children only;
For thy undaunted mettle should compose
Nothing but males.

Macbeth

O dearest soul: your cause doth strike my heart
With pity that doth make me sick!

Cymbeline

Lay not that flattering unction to your soul.

Hamlet

O, learn'd indeed were the astronomer
That knew the stars as I [know your] characters;
He'd lay the future open.

Cymbeline

The truest poetry is the most feigning, and lovers are
given to poetry.

As You Like It

You do not understand yourself so clearly.

Hamlet

Most miserable
Is the desire that's glorious.

Cymbeline

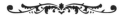

What a life is this,
That your poor friends must woo your company.

As You Like It

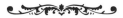

I might have look'd upon my queen's full eyes,
Have taken treasure from her lips, and left them
More rich for what they yielded.

The Winter's Tale

Why are you grown so rude? What change is this?

A Midsummer Night's Dream

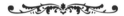

Love will not be spurred to what it loathes.

The Two Gentlemen of Verona

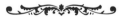

Heavens know some men are much to blame.

Cymbeline

You are full of pretty answers.

As You Like It

You think that none but your sheets are privy to your wishes.

Antony and Cleopatra

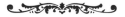

Love is your master, for he masters you;
And he that is so yoked by a fool
Methinks should not be chronicled for wise.

The Two Gentlemen of Verona

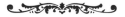

O, how bitter a thing it is to look into happiness through another man's eyes!

As You Like It

You put me off with limber vows.

The Winter's Tale

❧

Men are April when they woo, December when they wed.

As You Like It

❧

Now for the love of Love and her soft hours,
Let's not confound the time with conference harsh.

Antony and Cleopatra

❧

Wherefore was I to this keen mockery born?
When at your hands did I deserve this scorn?

A Midsummer Night's Dream

As an unperfect actor on the stage
Who with his fear is put besides his part,
Or some fierce thing replete with too much rage,
Whose strength's abundance weakens his own heart.
So I, for fear of trust, forget to say
The perfect ceremony of love's rite,
And in mine own love's strength seem to decay,
O'ercharged with burden of mine own love's might.
O, let my books be then the eloquence
And dumb presagers of my speaking breast,
Who plead for love and look for recompense
More than that tongue that more hath more express'd.
O, learn to read what silent love hath writ:
To hear with eyes belongs to love's fine wit.

Sonnet XXIII

Do not scorn me . . .
Say that you love me not, but say not so
In bitterness.

As You Like It

What is it to be false?
. . . if sleep charge Nature,
To break it with a fearful dream . . .
And cry myself awake?

Cymbeline

Love is merely a madness, and I tell you, deserves as
well a dark house and a whip as madmen do.

As You Like It

You dote on her that cares not for your love.

The Two Gentlemen of Verona

I know not how to tell thee who I am.

Romeo and Juliet

Come, come you are a fool,
And turn'd into the extremity of love.

As You Like It

Is whispering nothing?
I leaning cheek to cheek? Is meeting noses?
Kissing with inside lip? Stopping the career
Of laughter with a sigh?

The Winter's Tale

The oath of a lover is no stronger than the word
of a tapster. They are both the confirmer of false
reckonings.

As You Like It

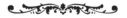

I shun the fire, for fear of burning.

The Two Gentlemen of Verona

I will not poison thee with my attaint,
Nor fold my fault in cleanly-coin'd excuses;
My sable ground of sin I will not paint,
To hide the truth of this false night's abuses:
My tongue shall utter all; mine eyes, like sluices,
As from a mountain-spring that feeds a dale,
Shall gush pure streams to purge my impure tale.

The Rape of Lucrece

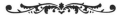

Maids are May when they are maids, but the sky
changes when they are wives.

As You Like It

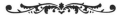

I am sick still. Heart-sick.

Cymbeline

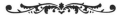

She was a woman, and was turned into a cold fish for
she would not exchange flesh with one that loved her.

The Winter's Tale

It is as easy to count atomies as to resolve the propositions of a lover.

As You Like It

I do forgive thee, unnatural though thou art.

The Tempest

It boots thee not
To be in love; where scorn is bought with groans;
Coy looks, with heart-sore sighs; one fading
moment's mirth, with twenty watchful, weary, tedious
nights.

The Two Gentlemen of Verona

If thy love were ever like to mine,
As sure I thinks did ever man love so,
How many actions most ridiculous
Hast thou been drawn to by thy fantasy?

As You Like It

I have bought the mansion of love
But not possess'd it.

Romeo and Juliet

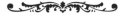

O hateful hands, to tear such loving;
Injurious wasps, to feed on such sweet honey,
And kill the bees that yield it, with your stings.

The Two Gentlemen of Verona

I beseech you, punish me not with your hard
thoughts.

As You Like It

Alack, alack, that heaven should practise stratagems
Upon so soft a subject as myself.

Romeo and Juliet

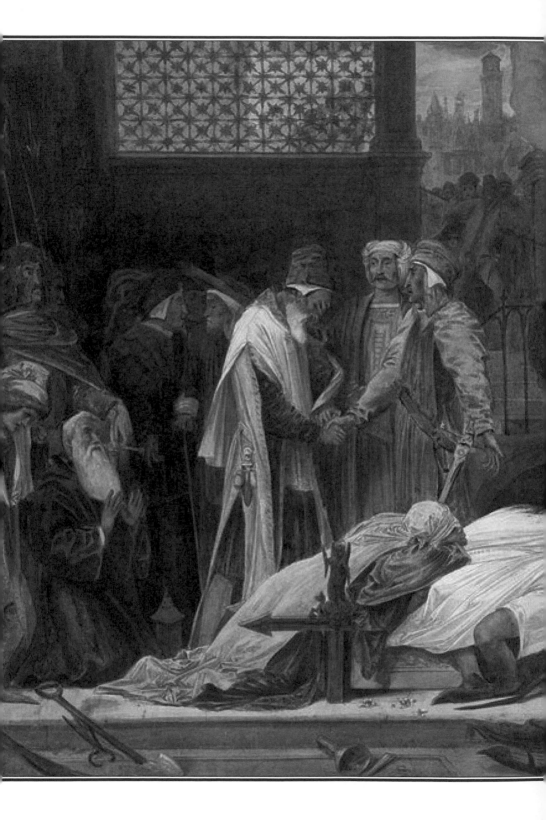

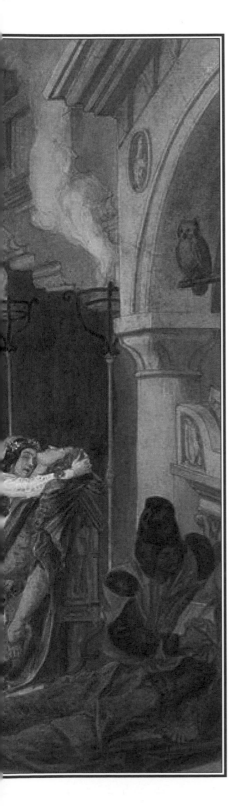

Lovers' Parting

Farewell, mad wench: you have a simple wit.

Love's Labour's Lost

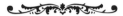

I shall be loved when I am lacked.

Coriolanus

Oft did she heave her napkin to her eyne . . .

A Lover's Complaint

I would not from thee.

Troilus and Cressida

'Tis almost morning, I would have thee gone,
And yet no farther than a wanton's bird,
that lets it hop a little from his hand
Like a poor prisoner in his twisted gyves,
And with a silken thread plucks it back again,
So loving-jealous of his liberty.

Romeo and Juliet

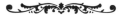

Men have died from time to time and worms have
eaten them, but not for love.

As You Like It

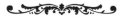

He fumbles up into a loose adieu,
And scants us with a single famish'd kiss
Distasted with the salt of broken tears.

Troilus and Cressida

But fare you well; perforce I must confess
I thought you lord of more true gentleness.

A Midsummer Night's Dream

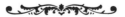

O think'st thou we shall ever meet again?

Romeo and Juliet

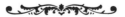

And you part so, mistress, I would I might never draw
sword again.

Twelfth Night

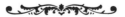

But, O my sweet, what labour is't to leave.

A Lover's Complaint

I have charged thee not to haunt about my doors.

Othello

A thousand times good night.

Romeo and Juliet

Hereafter, in a better world than this,
I shall desire more love and knowledge of you.

As You Like It

So sweet a kiss the golden sun gives not
To those fresh morning drops upon the rose,
As thy eye-beams when their fresh rays have smote
The night of dew that on my cheeks down flows.

Love's Labour's Lost

Good night: I'll be your fool no more.

Troilus and Cressida

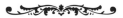

Have done: some grief shows much of love,
But much of grief shows still some want of wit.

Romeo and Juliet

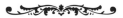

What, gone without a word?
Ay, so true love should do: it cannot speak,
For truth hath better deeds than words to grace it.

The Two Gentlemen of Verona

Thus can my love excuse the slow offence
Of my dull bearer when from thee I speed:
From where thou art why should I haste me thence?
Till I return, of posting is no need.
O, what excuse will my poor beast then find,
When swift extremity can seem but slow?
Then should I spur, though mounted on the wind;
In winged speed no motion shall I know:
Then can no horse with my desire keep pace;
Therefore desire of perfect'st love being made,
Shall neigh—no dull flesh—in his fiery race;
But love, for love, thus shall excuse my jade;
Since from thee going he went wilful-slow,
Towards thee I'll run, and give him leave to go.

Sonnet LI

Sweet, good night,
This bud of love, by summer's ripening breath,
May prove a beauteous flower when next we meet.

Romeo and Juliet

But come what may, I do adore thee so,
That danger shall seem sport, and I will go.

Twelfth Night

Be free, and fare thou well.

The Tempest

Farewell.
I will omit no opportunity
That may convey my greetings, love, to thee.

Romeo and Juliet

Fare thee well, thou art a gallant youth.

As You Like It

Bless you, fair shrew.

Twelfth Night

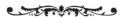

I have more care to stay than will to go.

Romeo and Juliet

O heaven, were man
But constant, he were perfect. That one error
Fills him with faults, makes him run though all th'
sins.

The Two Gentlemen of Verona

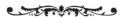

Some griefs are med'cinable
For it doth physic love.

Cymbeline

Go, girl, seek happy nights to happy days.

Romeo and Juliet

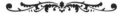

I warrant thou art a merry fellow, and car'st for nothing.

Twelfth Night

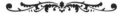

I should have been a woman.

As You Like It

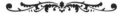

Good night, good night. As sweet repose and rest
Come to thy heart as that within my breast.

Romeo and Juliet

O, how this spring of love resembleth
The uncertain glory of an April day,
Which now shows all the beauty of the sun,
And by and by a cloud takes all away.

The Two Gentlemen of Verona

***

Good night, good night. Parting is such sweet sorrow
That I shall say good night til be marrow.

Romeo and Juliet

***

"For shame," he cries, "let go, and let me go;
My day's delight is past, my horse is gone,
And 'tis your fault I am bereft him so:
I pray you hence, and leave me here alone;
For all my mind, my thought, my busy care,
Is how to get my palfrey from the mare."

Venus and Adonis

You are too young in this.

As You Like It

❧

Alas, how love can trifle with itself.

The Two Gentlemen of Verona

❧

I am as fair now as I was erewhile.
Since night you lov'd me; yet since night you left me.

A Midsummer Night's Dream

❧

Can I go forward when my heart is here?

Romeo and Juliet

Write my queen,
And with mine eyes I'll drink the words you send,
Though ink be made of gall.

Cymbeline

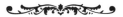

Make the doors upon a woman's wit, and it will out at
the casement; shut that, and 'twill out at the keyhole;
stop that, 'twill fly with the smoke out at the chimney.

As You Like It

O, 'tis the curse in love, and still approv'd,
When women cannot love where they're belov'd.

The Two Gentlemen of Verona

Thou shall be free as mountain winds.

The Tempest

Lovers' Parting

I pray you do not fall in love with me,
For I am falser than vows made in wine.
Besides, I like you not.

As You Like It

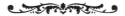

Alas, this parting strikes poor lovers dumb.

The Two Gentlemen of Verona

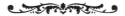

You shall hear from me still. The time shall not
Outgo my thinking on you.

Antony and Cleopatra

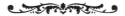

If sight and shape be true,
Why then my love adieu.

As You Like It

Now I see
The myst'ry of your loneliness.

All's Well That Ends Well

I would to heaven I had your potency.

Love's Labour's Lost

[Since] you be so tardy, come no more in my sight. I
had as life be wooed of a snail.

As You Like It

The kiss you take is better than you give;
Therefore, no kiss.

Troilus and Cressida

I see thou lov'st me not with the full weight that I love thee.

As You Like It

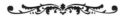

For in revenge of my contempt of Love,
Love hath chas'd sleep from my enthralled eyes,
And made them watchers of mine own heart's sorrow.

The Two Gentlemen of Verona

I'll tarry no longer with you. Farewell good Signor Love.

As You Like It

Do you love me, Master? No?

The Tempest

You have bereft me of all words, lady.

Troilus and Cressida

Let me hear of thee by letters.

The Two Gentlemen of Verona

Do you not know I am a woman? When I think, I must speak.

As You Like It

They do not love that do not show their love.

The Two Gentlemen of Verona

The boy disdains me,
He leaves me, scorns me: briefly die their joys
That place them on the truth of girls and boys.

Cymbeline

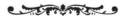

O thou that dost inhabit my breast,
Leave not the mansion so long tenantless,
Lest growing ruinous, the building fall,
And leave no memory of what it was.
Repair me, with thy presence.

The Two Gentlemen of Verona

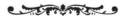

Laugh and let me go.

As You Like It

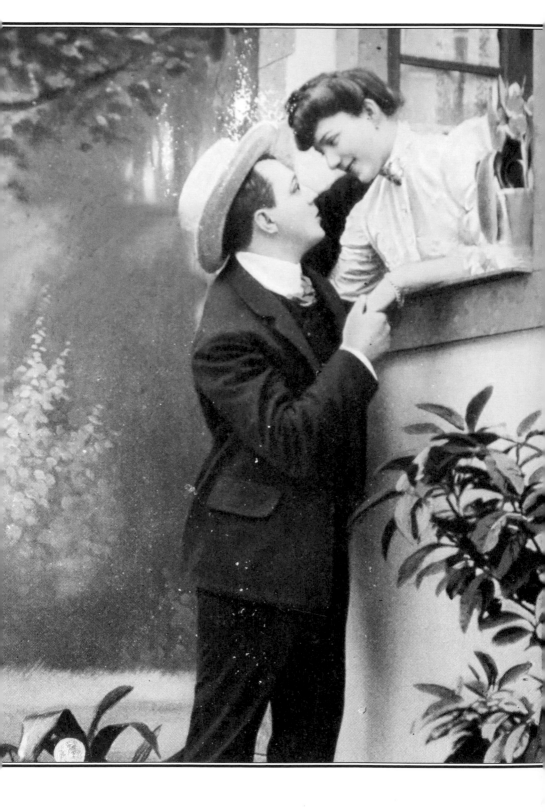

Love's Reconciliations

In sooth, I know not why I am so sad:
It wearies me; you say it wearies you;
But how I caught it, found it, or came by it,
What stuff 'tis made of, whereof it is born,
I am to learn;
And such a want-wit sadness makes of me,
That I have much ado to know myself.

The Merchant of Venice

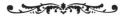

One word in private with you ere I die.

Love's Labour's Lost

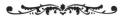

Thou art thyself.

Romeo and Juliet

This discipline shows thou hast been in love.

The Two Gentlemen of Verona

Thou look'st like one I lov'd indeed.

Pericles

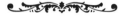

Give me your hand
And let me all your fortunes understand.

As You Like It

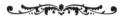

Love wrought these miracles.

The Taming of the Shrew

Thou art as wise as thou art beautiful.

A Midsummer Night's Dream

Take up the sword again, or take up me.

Richard III

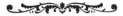

Thy face is mine.

Romeo and Juliet

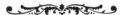

For my sake wear this,
It is a manacle of love, I'll place it
Upon this fairest prisoner.

Cymbeline

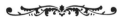

But, for my part,
I love him not, nor hate him not; and yet
I have more cause to hate him than to love him.

As You Like It

Shall I command thy love? I may. Shall I enforce
thy love?
I could. Shall I entreat thy love? I will.

Love's Labour's Lost

I have an interest in thy heart's proceeding.

Romeo and Juliet

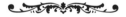

Fair glass of light, I lov'd you, and could still.

Pericles

Mistress, look on me,
Behold the window of my heart, mine eye,
What humble suit attends thy answer there;
Impose some service on me for thy love.

Love's Labour's Lost

And then end life when I end loyalty.

A Midsummer Night's Dream

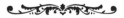

I prithee tell me what you think of me.

Twelfth Night

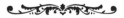

No more be grieved at that which thou hast done:
Roses have thorns, and silver fountains mud;
Clouds and eclipses stain both moon and sun,
And loathsome canker lives in sweetest bud.

Sonnet XXXV

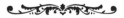

Had I brought hither a corrupted mind.
Thy speech had altered it.

Pericles

You are a thousand times a properer man
Than she is a woman.

As You Like It

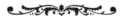

And now, what's the news with you?

Hamlet

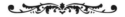

I do constantly believe you.

Love's Labour's Lost

How is it my soul, let's talk.

Romeo and Juliet

We that are true lovers run into strange capers; but as all is mortal in nature, so is all nature in love mortal in folly.

As You Like It

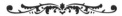

I will believe you by the syllable.

Pericles

Didst thou but know the only touch of love,
Thou wouldst as soon go kindle fire with snow
As seek to quench the fire of love with words.

The Two Gentlemen of Verona

They say the best men are moulded out of faults,
And, for the most, become much more the better
For being a little bad.

Measure for Measure

For which of my bad parts didst thou first fall in love
with me?

Much Ado About Nothing

I have no other but a woman's reason:
I think so, because I think so.

The Two Gentlemen of Verona

They say many young gentlemen flock to [you]
every day.

As You Like It

Madam, this service I have done for you
(Though you respect not aught your servant doth)
To hazard life, and rescue you from him
That would have forc'd your honor and your love.

The Two Gentlemen of Verona

O my dear lord, I crave no other, nor no better man.

Love's Labour's Lost

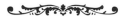

By my troth, you are very well met; by your leave, good mistress.

The Merry Wives of Windsor

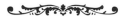

I am beholding to you for your sweet music this last night.

Pericles

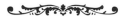

I wish but for the thing I have.

Romeo and Juliet

Give me thy hand.

Twelfth Night

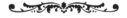

I love you now, but till now not so much.

Troilus and Cressida

Scorn at first makes after-love the more.

The Two Gentlemen of Verona

[Your] advice hath often still'd my brawling discontent.

Love's Labour's Lost

In thy youth thou wast as true a lover
As ever sigh'd upon a pillow.

As You Like It

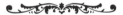

Noble mistress; 'tis fresh morning with me
When you are by at night.

The Tempest

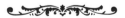

O, what a beast I was to chide . . .

Romeo and Juliet

My bosom, as a bed,
Shall lodge thee til thy wound be thoroughly heal'd.

The Two Gentlemen of Verona

Walk with me: speak freely.

Cymbeline

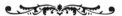

Swear by thy gracious self,
Which is the god of my idolatry,
And I'll believe thee.

Romeo and Juliet

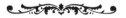

Do you love me?

The Tempest

Hear me, my love: be thou but true of heart.

Troilus and Cressida

A thousand oaths, an ocean of tears,
And instances of infinite of love,
Warrant . . . welcome.

The Two Gentlemen of Verona

In following [you] I follow but myself.

Othello

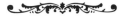

I do remember . . .
Some lively touches.

As You Like It

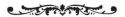

A woman sometimes scorns what best contents her.

The Two Gentlemen of Verona

By my modesty,
The jewel in my dower, I would not wish
Any companion in the world but you.

The Tempest

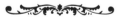

O infinite virtue! Com'st thou smiling from
The world's great snare uncaught?

Antony and Cleopatra

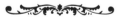

Here is my hand, for my true constancy.

The Two Gentlemen of Verona

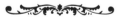

Sweet, above thought I love thee.

Troilus and Cressida

Jove I thank thee, I will smile, I will do every thing
that thou wilt have me.

Twelfth Night

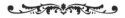

You have the grace by your fair prayer
To soften . . .

Love's Labour's Lost

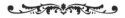

I'll give no blemish to [your] honor, none.

The Winter's Tale

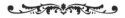

My duty, madam, and most humble service.

Twelfth Night

Though I lov'd you well, I woo'd you not.

Troilus and Cressida

Thou chid'st me oft . . .
For doting, not for loving.

Romeo and Juliet

I am a fool to weep at what I am glad of.

The Tempest

Pardon me, or strike me, if you please;
I cannot be much lower than my knees.

Pericles

Shall I abide
In this dull world, which in thy absence is
No better than a sty?

Antony and Cleopatra

Upon my knees,
I charm you, by my once-commended beauty,
By all your vows of love and that great vow
Which did incorporate and make us one.
That you unfold to me, yourself, your half,
Why you are heavy?

Julius Caesar

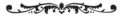

Plight me the full assurance of your faith,
That my most jealous and too doubtful soul
May live at peace.

Twelfth Night

Fair thoughts be your fair pillow.

Troilus and Cressida

Vouchsafe to wear this ring.

Richard III

I would I knew [thy] mind.

The Two Gentlemen of Verona

I will be more jealous of thee than a Barbary cock-pigeon over his hen, more clamorous than a parrot against rain, more new-fangled than an ape, more giddy in my desires than a monkey.

As You Like It

There's nothing ill can dwell in such a temple.

The Tempest

If that thy bent of love be honorable,
Thy purpose marriage, send me word tomorrow . . .
Where and at what time thou wilt perform the rite.

Romeo and Juliet

You are such a woman, a man knows not at what ward
you lie.

Troilus and Cressida

It pleaseth me so well, that I will see you wed;
And then, with what haste you can, get you to bed.

Pericles

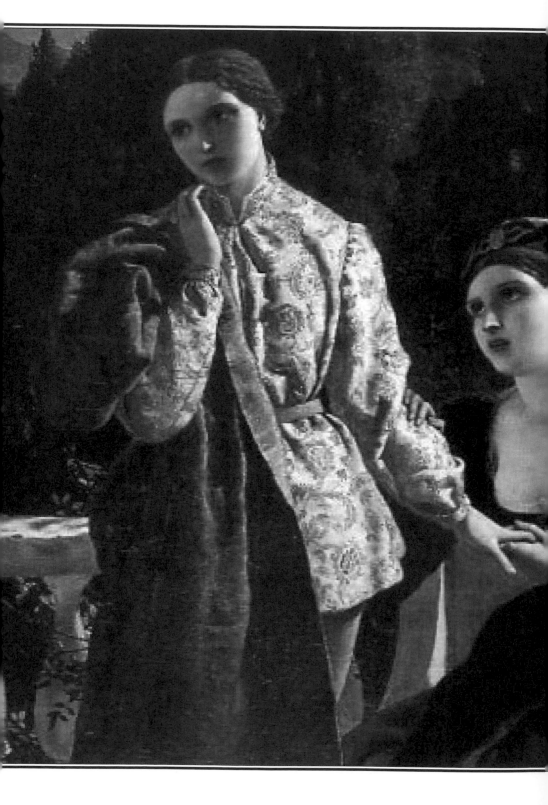

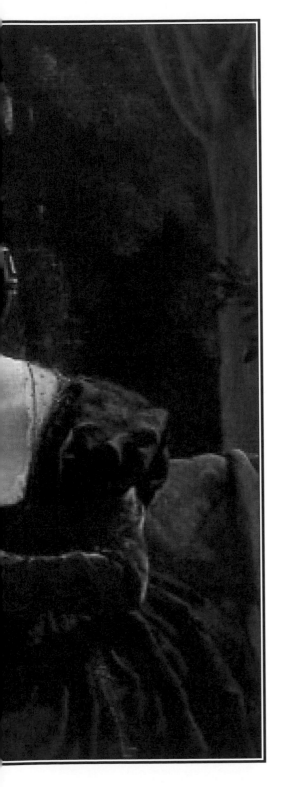

The Hope of Love

Now can I break my fast, dine, sup and sleep
Upon the very naked name of Love.

The Two Gentlemen of Verona

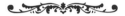

Let me live here ever.

Romeo and Juliet

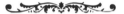

Go to your bosom,
Knock there, and ask your heart what it doth know.

Love's Labour's Lost

It is ten times true, for truth is truth
To th'end of reck'ning.

Measure for Measure

Were't not affection chains thy tender days
To the sweet glances of thy honour'd love,
I rather would entreat thy company
To see the wonders of the world abroad.

The Two Gentlemen of Verona

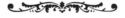

Love is a smoke made with the fume of sighs;
Being purg'd, a fire sparkling in lovers' eyes;
Being vex'd, a sea nourish'd with lovers' tears;
What is it else? A madness most discreet,
A choking gall, and a preserving sweet.

Romeo and Juliet

Heaven that I had thy head!

Pericles

I am a friend, and one that knows you well.

Romeo and Juliet

I see how thine eye would emulate the diamond.

Love's Labour's Lost

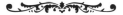

Our praises are our wages.

The Winter's Tale

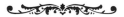

Live a little, comfort a little cheer thyself a little.

As You Like It

Would I might but ever see [this] man!

The Tempest

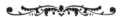

[Thou] wear the rose
Of youth upon [you].

Antony and Cleopatra

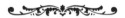

Well, or ill, I am bound to you.

Cymbeline

Our love and comforts should increase
Even as our days do grow.

Othello

The Hope of Love

Were I were young, for your sake.

The Merry Wives of Windsor

❧

Love talks with better knowledge, and knowledge
with dearer love.

Measure for Measure

❧

Though, Fortune, visible an enemy,
Should chase us . . . power no jot
Hath she to change our loves.

The Winter's Tale

❧

I shall here abide . . . comforted . . . that there is this
jewel in the world that I may see again.

Cymbeline

For [your] bounty,
There was no winter in't; an autumn it was
That grew the more by reaping.

Antony and Cleopatra

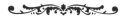

Love's a mighty lord.
And hath so humbled me, as I confess
There is no woe to this correction,
Nor to his service, no such joy on earth.

The Two Gentlemen of Verona

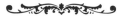

I will follow thee to the last gasp with truth and
loyalty.

As You Like It

Nobly yoke
A smiling with a sigh; as if the sigh
Was that it was, for not being such a smile.

Cymbeline

Thou and I are too wise to woo peaceably.

Much Ado About Nothing

We [are] as twinn'd lambs that . . . frisk i'th'sun,
And bleat the one at th'other.

The Winter's Tale

I leave myself, my friends, and all, for love.

The Two Gentlemen of Verona

I will remain the loyal'st husband that e'er did plight troth.

Cymbeline

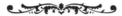

You are my true and honourable wife,
As dear to me as are the ruddy drops
That visit my sad heart.

Julius Caesar

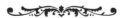

How beauteous mankind is!

The Tempest

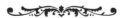

They say we are
Almost as like as eggs.

The Winter's Tale

Let what is here contain'd relish of love.

Cymbeline

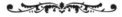

Lift up thy countenance, as it were the day
Of celebration of that nuptial which
We two have sworn shall come.

The Winter's Tale

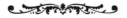

On a love-book pray for my success.

The Two Gentlemen of Verona

Lead me on.

Twelfeth Night

[Love is] but a folly bought with wit,
Or else a wit by folly vanquished.

The Two Gentlemen of Verona

Come, here's my heart.

Cymbeline

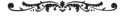

Thou shalt be worshipp'd, kiss'd, lov'd, and ador'd.

The Two Gentlemen of Verona

I am yours forever.

The Winter's Tale

The sight of lovers feedth those in love.

As You Like It

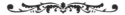

Love is blind. O, that you had mine eyes, or your own eyes had the lights they were wont to have.

The Two Gentlemen of Verona

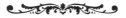

[Thy] beauty claims
No worse a husband than the best of men.

Antony and Cleopatra

Since thou lov'st, love still, and thrive therein,
Even as I would, when I to love begin.

The Two Gentlemen of Verona

Now I think on thee,
My hunger's gone: but even before, I was
At point to sink, for food.

Cymbeline

Upon a homely object, Love can wink.

The Two Gentlemen of Verona

You were better speak first, and when you were graveled for lack of matter, you might take occasion to kiss.

As You Like It

Age cannot wither, nor custom stale [your] infinite variety.

Antony and Cleopatra

Now, no discourse, except it be of love.

The Two Gentlemen of Verona

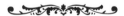

You may ride's
With one soft kiss a thousand furlongs ere
With spur we heat an acre.

The Winter's Tale

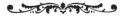

I do applaud thy spirit.

The Two Gentlemen of Verona

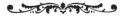

Let your fair eyes and gentle wishes go with me.

As You Like It

Boy thou hast look'd thyself into my grace,
And art mine own.

Cymbeline

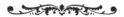

When it stands well with him, it stands well with her.

The Two Gentlemen of Verona

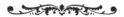

Heaven knows how I love you, and you shall one day
find it.

The Merry Wives of Windsor

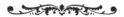

Nothing but fair is that which you inherit.

Love's Labour's Lost

Upon [thy] brow shame is asham'd to sit.

Romeo and Juliet

My master and my lord!

Antony and Cleopatra

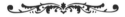

I would you were as I would have you be.

Twelfth Night

Better a little chiding than a great deal of heartbreak.

The Merry Wives of Windsor

If music be the food of love, play on,
Give me excess if it, that, surfeiting,
The appetite may sicken, and so die.

Twelfth Night

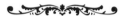

I will marry upon any reasonable demands.

The Merry Wives of Windsor

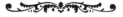

Hang there my verse, in witness of my love.

As You Like It

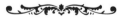

And what love can do, that dares love attempt.

Romeo and Juliet

I will tell thee wonders.

Love's Labour's Lost

All happiness bechance to thee.

The Two Gentlemen of Verona

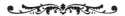

O, that you were yourself! but, love, you are
No longer yours than you yourself here live:
Against this coming end you should prepare,
And your sweet semblance to some other give.

Sonnet XIII

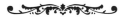

. . . If love be blind,
It best agrees with night.

Romeo and Juliet

Let there come a tempest of provocation, I will shelter me here.

The Merry Wives of Windsor

Though to myself forsworn, to thee I'll faithful prove.

Love's Labour's Lost

Hence, bashful cunning!
And prompt me plain and holy innocence!
I am your wife if you will marry me;
If not, I'll die your maid: to be your fellow
You may deny me; but I'll be your servant,
Whether you will or no.

The Tempest

Come what sorrow can,
It cannot countervail the exchange of joy
That one short minute gives me in [thy] sight.

Romeo and Juliet

The Hope of Love

Come temperate nymphs, and help to celebrate
A contract of true love; be not too late.

The Tempest

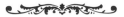

Shall I compare thee to a summer's day?
Thou art more lovely and more temperate:
Rough winds do shake the darling buds of May,
And summer's lease hath all too short a date:
Sometime too hot the eye of heaven shines,
And often is his gold complexion dimm'd;
And every fair from fair sometime declines,
By chance or nature's changing course untrimm'd;
But thy eternal summer shall not fade
Nor lose possession of that fair thou owest;
Nor shall Death brag thou wander'st in his shade,
When in eternal lines to time thou growest:
So long as men can breathe or eyes can see,
So long lives this and this gives life to thee.

Sonnet XVIII

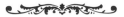

I do not doubt thy faith.

Pericles

I cannot be
Mine own, nor anything to any, if
I be not thine.

The Winter's Tale

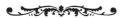

You did not know
How much you were my conqueror, and that
My sword, made weak by my affection, would
Obey it in all cause.

Antony and Cleopatra

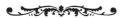

When he shall die
Take him and cut him out in little stars,
And he will make the face of heaven so fine
That all the world will be in love with night,
And pay no worship to the garish sun.

Romeo and Juliet

I have great comfort from this fellow.

The Tempest

If knowledge be the mark, to know thee shall suffice.

Love's Labour's Lost

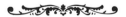

Love knows I love;
But who?
Lips, do not move,
No man must know.

Twelfth Night

Beautiful tyrant, fiend angelical,
Dove-feather'd raven, wolvish-ravening lamb!

Romeo and Juliet

Albeit I will confess thy father's wealth
Was the first motive that I woo'd thee . . .
Yet, wooing thee, I found thee of more value
Than stamps in gold or sums in sealed bags;
And 'tis the very riches of thyself
That now I am at.

The Merry Wives of Windsor

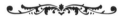

My sweet mistress
Weeps when she see's me work.

The Tempest

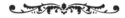

Come, madam wife, sit by my side
And let the world slip, we shall ne'er be younger.

The Taming of the Shrew

He loves you well that holds his life of you.

Pericles

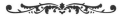

I would I knew thy heart.

Richard III

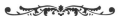

The sweetest honey
Is loathsome in his own deliciousness,
And in the taste confounds the appetite.
Therefore love moderately; long love doth so.

Romeo and Juliet

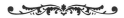

I bequeath a happy peace to you.

Pericles

I love thee, by my life I do;
I swear by that which I will lose for thee
To prove him false that says I love thee not.

A Midsummer Night's Dream

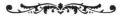

So dying love lives still.

Troilus and Cressida

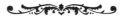

Dost thou love me? I know thou wilt say "Ay,"
And I will take thy word.

Romeo and Juliet

Come . . . we'll to bed.

The Taming of the Shrew